Your 5:2 Diet Days:
Tasty Recipes for One

Lucy Lonsdale

ISBN-13: 978-1482648393

To my son Joel

For his boundless enthusiasm for these recipes

Author's note:

Every care has been taken in checking all the information presented in this book. However, human error can creep in anywhere without warning, so I cannot accept responsibility for any mistakes that are discovered.

Contents

                              Page

Weighing Up The 5:2 Diet   5

On a Personal Note...   15

Using This Book   16

Daily Menus   23

Index of Meals   76

Weighing Up The 5:2 Diet

What is the 5:2 Diet?

Put very simply, this increasingly popular diet is a way of eating that involves choosing any two non-consecutive days each week and restricting your total calories intake on those days to no more than 500 calories for women or 600 for men. For the other five days you can follow your normal diet.

How does this diet differ from any other one out there?

It differs in that you only have to follow it for two days a week, unlike other diets which entail changing the way you eat on a daily basis. It does not make you envious of someone who is tucking in to your favourite high fat, calorie-laden foods, since you know that on the other five days you also have that choice. And, as well as losing weight, there seem to be other health benefits and good reasons to adopt this intermittent form of calorie restriction.

What are the benefits of the 5:2 Diet?

Steady weight loss, which is virtually guaranteed if you are following this diet, is only one of the advantages even though it is clearly an important one and the one that attracts most people to it in the first place. But it is said that it also protects against developing some brain diseases such as Alzheimer's and Parkinson's. In addition, there are claims that it lowers unhealthy cholesterol levels, normalizes blood glucose, raises your energy levels after a short while and helps you to live longer. And if those are not sufficient reasons to give it a try, it is worth considering the claim that this diet also affords protection from developing heart disease, type 2 diabetes and cancer.

That sounds impressive, but what evidence is there that this diet really does have these benefits?

This is an interesting and somewhat more complex question. There has been great deal of research with rodents but comparatively few studies with humans. The Institute of Aging, in Baltimore, Maryland, USA, conducted controlled studies with mice that showed definitively that the ones who were fed the 5:2 way lived longer in mice years than the group who were fed normally. They also showed a far slower decline in brain function than the other mice. Additionally, they appeared more energetic and active than their fellow mice and displayed a markedly lower tendency to develop the sort of other diseases mentioned above. Whilst all this is very promising we cannot be certain that human beings will respond in precisely the same way.

However, I don't want to give the impression that I am anything less than enthusiastic about this diet which many people are finding very helpful, as indeed I am myself. Research with the mice is a useful indicator that for most of us, this diet could well prove to be the best way forward for eating our way to considerably longer, healthier lives.

Only long term scientifically reliable, controlled studies with a significant number of people will give us the answers we seek. For the time being there is an enormous amount of anecdotal evidence from people who have tried and stayed on the diet for several months. So we have enough information already to make our own informed decision about embarking on this diet; and our own experience will tell us whether it suits us and if, or how, we want to use it in the long term.

I have heard the Laron Syndrome mentioned in connection with the 5:2 Diet. What is it?

In a village in Ecuador there is a group of around a hundred villagers who have Laron's syndrome (named after Zvi Laron, an Israeli researcher who first reported this condition in the nineteen sixties). They have been scientifically studied over a period of twenty-two years to find out why, barring alcoholism and accidents, they were living much longer lives than any of the other villagers. The reason seems to be that they have a genetic lack of the IGF 1 growth hormone which is responsible for childhood growth. This hormone lack accounts for why people in this group are unusually small - usually less than three and a half feet tall.

So unusual and rare is the syndrome worldwide (affecting about three hundred people in total) that it has attracted much interest from scientists who have studied the villagers and others with this syndrome and then applied their findings to animal research.

Those with Laron's syndrome in the Ecuadorian village do not diet, some smoke and they all eat whatever food they want. Yet despite leading what we might consider very unhealthy lives and some becoming obese, they do not develop many of the usual serious illnesses like diabetes, cancer, heart disease and onset of brain diseases such as dementia, associated with age. They also look much younger for longer and generally live to a greater age than those without this syndrome. If they ate more healthily and did not smoke they would probably live even longer but knowing they have this immunity tends to make them carefree rather than focus on living a hundred years or more.

Ok, but what has this got to do with the 5:2 diet specifically?

It has been discovered that the IGF 1 hormone, essential whilst we are growing into adults, can work against us once we begin to age. High amounts of it appear to cause damage to cells, which leads to a greater susceptibility to developing serious health problems. This in turn lowers our quality of life as well as shortening it considerably. Restricting calorie intake on the two days a week, as in the 5:2 diet, causes a lowering of the level of the insulin-like IGF1 hormone, kick-starting our bodies into switching on DNA repair genes and focusing on the essential reparation of existing damaged cells instead of making new ones.

It seems like following this diet is a brilliant way to ensure that our bodies can undo the harm already done to cells and reverse some potentially serious effects of the aging process.

This sounds good so far but is it a safe diet to follow?

I have consulted a number of medical doctors about this and all of them tell me that, as long as the diet is followed sensibly (not becoming obsessive over calorie-counting, keeping it to two, non-consecutive days per week and eating a normal diet on the other five days), it cannot harm, and could possibly be very beneficial. Some of them have, in fact, started this diet themselves!

Are there any reasons why anyone should not go on this diet?

Yes, it is definitely not suitable for children, pregnant or breast-feeding women, diabetics, or someone with an eating disorder. Furthermore, if you have any serious health problem or are in doubt about whether this form of eating is suitable for you, it is very important that you consult your GP before making a decision.

Some nutritionists have expressed worries that food restriction carries a danger of developing eating disorders. Could this happen?

Being obsessive about any form of dieting can trigger an eating disorder. As far as the 5:2 diet is concerned, 'starvation' and 'fasting' are words that have been used by some to describe the two days of calorie restriction. If these terms are taken literally (i.e. no food whatsoever) then someone could develop anorexia, especially if they then began also to severely restrict calorie intake for the rest of the week. Likewise, it is possible to become bulimic if, after each low calorie day, a person starts binge eating.

It's really about taking a sensible approach and not allowing food (or the lack of it) to become the central focus of your entire life.

The 5:2 diet carries an extremely low risk for the majority of people becoming eating-disordered, probably less so than in the case of many other, more faddish diets. That is, of course, provided it is tackled with a large dose of common sense and does not totally exclude any important groups of food that our bodies need. A particular advantage of this particular way of eating is that no food is completely banned.

But isn't binge eating a realistic possibility the day after consuming only a quarter of the normal daily calorie amount?

On the face of it you would think that this could well happen. It's understandable to assume that restricting calorie intake on one day would lead to gorging on food the next. However, we are creatures of habit and, surprising as it might seem, tend to revert to our normal eating patterns. This has certainly been the case for the majority on this diet. Even the scientists who have closely observed 5:2 dieters have been surprised by this fact.

It's not difficult to start a diet with enthusiasm but how easy is it to stick to this one?

I have spoken to many people who have had experience of trying out lots of diets – 'The cabbage soup diet', 'The Atkins diet', 'The morning banana diet' are a few that randomly spring to mind. Results with some of these were initially encouraging, with impressive weight loss whilst on them. But will power is a tricky thing and for all but a rare handful of mortals, persevering for a lengthy period with any regime that permanently denies them their favourite foods is too difficult.

On the 5:2 diet, on the other hand, you do not have to cut out any of the foods you like. Even if their calorie count is way too high to include in the low calorie days, you can enjoy them on the other five days of the week. This is probably the main reason that this particular diet is becoming increasingly popular. Many have started and, months later, are still on it. It's not a fad diet but rather a different way of eating. Not only do people on it see results quickly but they know that, even if they are finding it hard going, they have five other days a week that are as easy as they were before embarking on this diet and probably less guilt-ridden!

It does not become unmanageable when you only have to think about reducing your calories for two days in a week instead of struggling with cutting them down every single day! And since you decide which two days in the week are best for you as well as being able to alter them week by week according to your social schedule (you probably won't want to choose any day you're going out to a restaurant, for example), the choice is all yours. Each week may have a different two days or you may find it more convenient to keep to the same two. You are in control!

Is this a totally new concept?

Not at all. Way back in time our ancestors did not have three meals a day, fast food outlets or a great choice of supermarkets. They had to go out and hunt for food. So on some days they ate a feast, whilst on other days they ate very little unless they were exceptionally clever hunters with a lot of slow running animals nearby! Then, as time passed, people grew a lot of their food which meant that it wasn't plentiful all the time because it was seasonal. Later still, during World War Two and for some years after, food was rationed. Obesity was not a problem. It can't just be co-incidence that a large proportion of the UK population (post war baby boomers) are still alive and kicking! They were brought up on fresh food - many homes did not own a refrigerator until the fifties so meat, fruit and vegetables had to be bought daily or kept in a large cupboard, better known as a larder, for a few days.

Well, that's the history lesson over!

What if I finally find my weight is beginning to drop further than I wanted. Is that the time to stop?

No, because if you are fortunate enough to reach that stage you can simply drop to having one low calorie day per week to maintain your current healthy weight.

I enjoy cooking but on my low calorie days will I have to eat plain, boring foods and only a small amount of those?

On the contrary, as the recipes further on in this book will demonstrate, you can have fun cooking a good variety of colourful, interesting meals to suit your taste. These range from ones that are very easy and quick to prepare to some that involve more time and skill. The choice is yours!

What are things that I need to be aware of to help me to avoid the difficulties that this diet might throw up?

First off, less food intake on the low calorie days could lead to headaches. This is easily avoided by drinking plenty of water throughout the day, especially before a meal. Besides keeping you well-hydrated, water will help to stave off really uncomfortable hunger pangs and headaches and avoid constipation and fatigue. Generally we should be drinking around eight glasses daily anyway but an extra intake will help on low calorie days. It doesn't have to be boring either: green tea is full of healthy antioxidants, calorie free and provides an excellent way of increasing water intake. And since almost all of the major organs in our bodies depend on adequate water consumption, it is vital to drink sufficient.

Secondly, you may find it easier to reserve going to the gym, brisk walking, swimming or whatever your exercise of choice, for the five days of non-restriction of calories. Initially, you may find your energy levels dropping a little. Ultimately, however, you will probably find that you have more energy than usual, perhaps because your legs have less weight to support!.

Thirdly, although you may perhaps be tempted, it is unwise to weigh yourself daily, which could lead to obsession. Once a week is sufficient and will give you a pleasant surprise.

If you have any more questions about the 5:2 diet please free to email me at: lucylonsdale@hotmail.co.uk and I will do my very best to answer them.

On a Personal Note...

Until my early thirties I did not have a weight problem. I thought I was one of those lucky people who can eat whatever they like and still keep their weight at a steady healthy level. So it never occurred to me to go on a diet. I just didn't need to.

Six pregnancies later, neglecting to follow all the sensible advice about post natal exercises and ignoring my monthly gym membership (although every month began with a resolution to work out regularly), my lack of attention to my body was obvious to all, especially me! Every visible part of me had travelled south and my five foot two inch frame had ballooned to an unhealthy twelve and a half stone. That's more than three stone over my ideal weight!

I began the long, uncomfortable journey of yoyo dieting. Any and every new diet regime I came across was, initially, to be my route to an even sleeker, slimmer healthier body than I'd had in the first place. I started each one with religious zeal and determination to succeed, convincing myself each time that this was it! I'd found the only diet that worked and suited my lifestyle at the same time.

And so it began. I worked my way rapidly through them one by one. I won't bore you with the entire list but among them featured: the Hay, Acai Berry, the South Beach, Slim Fast, Gorgeously Green and the Lemon diets which were all-consuming for a week or two before I drifted back to my old well-trodden, familiar eating habits. And so the scales went up and down on a regular basis until I finally gave up! I concluded that I was one of many whose will power was strong initially but short-lived. Not only was I back to square one each time but I felt increasingly disheartened and began to worry a lot about my health.

I have now discovered that I am genetically pre-disposed to piling on the pounds, which is not to say that it's inevitable and that there is nothing I can do about it. I have to take responsibility for myself and cannot use that as an excuse. However, I do envy my husband who can eat whatever he fancies and who, just like all the relatives on his father's side, never puts on a dangerously unhealthy amount of weight. His father, uncles, aunts and grandparents all lived, or are living, long and productive lives.

They all had (or have) a brilliant sense of humour too, though whether or not there is any significance in that I don't know!

My mother was morbidly obese and all my aunts were way overweight. Unfortunately, the heaviness of the problem extended beyond their size leading to serious health problems like diabetes and heart disease.

If I wanted to see my children develop their careers and enjoy any future grandchildren and great-grandchildren, it was crystal clear that I had to pull my socks up (if I could reach them), find a way to lose weight and hopefully live a long, active healthy life.

It was at this crucial point that the 5:2 diet hit the scene in a big way. It sounded too good to be true but the only way I could possibly find out if this were the case would be to give it a go.

And so I began with earnest zeal, whilst my family waited patiently for yet another diet to bite the dust.

The first couple of weeks were quite difficult. I was just eating a couple of scrambled eggs with a piece of ham for breakfast and having grilled chicken or fish and vegetables for dinner. I missed out lunch, had headaches, felt very tired and hungry and lacked energy. And I was on the point of giving up yet again.

But I decided that it was now or never time and that I would think carefully before abandoning this diet. There was far too much at steak - sorry, stake...

My husband was adamant that he was not going on any diet with me so I had to try to make tasty meals for one. However, this became an interesting project, not just a time-consuming one. During the hours of the normal five days of the week I began to experiment with colours of various foods (the colours of different foods, when combined, not only look attractive but the more variation in the colours the greater the nutritional value on the plate). I spent hours researching the calorie content of ingredients for the recipes I was compiling and found that I was actually beginning to enjoy the process. I had never felt the slightest edge of happiness on any other diet.

I prepared in other ways ahead of my low calorie days - I had already decided to leave at least two days between them. I resolved to increase my water intake significantly. I began to list calorie free drinks and beverages low in calories so that I could give myself more options than just water for the two days. And, as I know the two low calorie days can be to suit yourself provided they are not consecutive, I settled on Mondays and Fridays as best for me. If I were to be invited to a wedding or a party, or should my husband decide we need a night out, then I could always shift the days around.

So by week three I had the beginnings of a plan and felt considerably more in control. I had a few recipes for my low calorie days which kept me busy and able to cope with brief feelings of hunger whilst looking forward to the meal I was preparing. When I told my daughter-in-law about some of the recipes she asked for copies. I was delighted when she rang me and said that she had prepared one of the lunches the night before and enjoyed it at work the following day. She was looking forward to doubling the quantities of a dinner recipe and cooking it in the evening for the two of them.

And that is how my recipe section in this book evolved over the ensuing weeks and months.

I discovered that apart from water there were a lot of other drinks that added few or even no calories: black tea, green tea, fruit infusions, beef extract, yeast extract...

I have now been practising the 5:2 diet religiously for six months, a feat I never thought possible. And I have joined the growing ranks of its fans. I have no more will power than I had before I started it but this time around I don't need to make a superhuman effort. It is a far easier diet than any I have ever attempted. I lost three and a half stone in total steadily over five months and feel so much lighter, in spirit as well as in body. It is like I've finally stopped constantly carrying around small child (roughly the same weight as I shed). To put that in another context, try lifting forty-nine pounds of shopping and then imagine that weight distributed around your body permanently!

For the past month I have been focusing on one low calorie day per week and found that the weight has not only stayed off but that my new healthy level remains fairly constant.

I have lots more energy, my mood has improved (ask my husband!), and I feel massively more motivated in so many ways. I am now able to exercise on a regular basis and join in more social activities than I have in ages.

On my five "normal" days I try to follow a healthy Mediterranean eating style with plenty of fruit, vegetables and the odd glass or two of red wine. I continue to enjoy an occasional slice of tasty cake and a small piece of dark chocolate now and then. I never feel deprived or guilty since I know that the 5:2 diet allows for any choice I may make (within reason, of course).

Perhaps the biggest surprise has been the fact that on my "normal" days I am less hungry than I used to be and have a considerably lower craving for sweet things.

I intend to continue this transformation of my eating habits for the foreseeable future. And, as if I needed any more evidence than I already have, my latest battery of blood tests results are the icing on the cake. I was taking a daily statin pill for twelve years because my cholesterol level was so high. I decided on a statin holiday three months ago, with my GP's approval, knowing that a few weeks off a statin for someone with no pre-existing heart disease was not a problem,. Now my doctor has taken me off them since I have a level well within the normal range. He has also confirmed that my blood glucose is normal and that I no longer run the risk of diabetes.

Having followed the 5:2 diet for a few months, get yourself medically assessed by your doctor to see how the diet is suiting you. We are all different and my own experience is not enough on which to base a decision for your future However, in time I hope (and expect) that like me you will feel lighter, healthier and happier.

Using This Book

As well as being an introduction to the 5:2 diet, this book's purpose is to provide a range of enjoyable, tasty, calorie-controlled menus for one person. When I started to follow this diet I spent a lot of time seeking out recipes that I could use myself. This was harder than you might imagine. Often I would encounter a dish that sounded delicious, only to read that it fed eight to ten people. Dividing ingredients by ten was not always practical – making a casserole for one person, for instance, is not easy unless you make more than you want and store or freeze the rest.

So I spent some time experimenting and adapting to find out what worked and tasted good for my meal and what didn't. The result is what follows in the next section. A couple of recipes make more than you will need at the time: the banana muffins, for instance. But in these cases the extra portions are ones that store easily – or that your nearest and dearest will eat even before they get that far! And doubling the amounts is easily done if you want to share a meal with someone else.

Of course, your entire calorie allowance can be used up in one meal or two. But I found that a three-meals-a-day regime suits me best, as I guess it will for many other people, and that is how I have set out the meals in this book.

Each calorie-restricted day is listed as a complete menu of three meals, scintillatingly entitled Menu One, Menu Two and so on. The calorie value for each meal is given as well as the day's total calories. I considered giving the calorie value for each ingredient but decided that this was impractical. After all, measuring a tablespoon of this or a cup of that is not an exact science and so there are variations built into the system already. And anyone searching the internet for calorific values of individual foods will soon be struck by the widely differing results they find. As an example, if you look up the calories for "1 slice wholemeal bread". What you will find depends on what brand of bread you look at, the size of each slice, etc – and what if you don't eat the crusts? So, as you can see, it would be a misleading for me to list the calorie count for every individual item. It's more relevant is that you keep to the amounts mentioned in the recipe. By all means read the information on the packaging but don't get obsessive about a few calories here or there. The meals as they stand obey the spirit of the 5:2 diet and that is what matters.

It would be virtually impossible to write a set of daily menus to suit everyone and I recognise that some of the menus may contain a meal here or there that may not be to your taste. To that end, I have listed all the breakfasts, lunches and dinners after the menu days, together with the calorie count of each one given in brackets. That should enable you to mix and match as you wish – simply make sure that your chosen meals add up to no more than 500 calories (or for a man, 600). If you happen to go over your target number by a few calories, don't panic – I've done it myself and I can assure you that it made no difference!

Almost all the ingredients listed are easily available – I've tried to steer clear of anything that might prove problematic to source. An ingredient that a few people may find difficult to obtain in the UK is the Edamame beans. I know that Waitrose and some healthfood shops stock them. In the USA they are being hailed as a superfood (as blueberries are) so they will probably arrive in the UK in a big way before long.

There was a time not so long ago when the sweet-toothed dieter was left with a rather unappealing choice: no sugar at all or artificial sweeteners. Mercifully, this is no longer the case. There are several natural sweeteners available that are low in calorific value and one that is completely calorie free, called stevia. This may sound like a trendy name for a baby girl but in fact it is an extract from the leaves of a plant of that name, which grows in North and South America. In the UK it is marketed under a number of brand names the easiest to find being Truvia. In the US the main brand appears to be Sweet Leaf. Having used stevia extract myself I can say that it tastes good and is completely free from the artificial overtones that characterise many other sweeteners. It is extremely sweet though, and should be used sparingly – a third of a teaspoon is equivalent to a full teaspoon of sugar!

Another very useful aid for the dieter comes in the form of a spray can (pump-action, not aerosol) of 1 calorie cooking oil, available as sunflower or olive oil. This delivers one calorie of oil per spray. I have found it very useful for frying eggs, making omelettes and indeed for any frying that doesn't require deep fat. About four sprays is sufficient to fry an egg. When you realise that a tablespoonful of olive oil contains 120 calories, the benefits of this spray become immediately obvious.

If your day's total on any day is below 500 (men read 600), you have the leeway to enjoy drinks with some calorie count. Tea taken black contains no calories, but add a splash of semi-skimmed milk and it rises to about 15. Using skimmed milk takes this down to 10 calories. These need to be factored into your day's total. To help you with drinks you might enjoy on a calorie-restricted day, I have compiled a list. It's worth noting that even within the zero-calorie list there is a reasonable choice.

Zero Calorie:
Still water, tap or bottled
Sparkling mineral water
Black tea
Earl Grey tea
Rooibos (Red Bush) tea
Green tea
Diet cola
Diet soda
Iced tea, black

There is a range of zero-rated flavoured canned drinks marketed under the brand name Zevia. Their website lists fifteen flavours. They apparently contain natural flavourings and no artificial sweeteners, using instead the previously-mentioned stevia extract. They are manufactured in the United States and at the time of writing are making their first appearance in the UK, though I have yet to try them. I am not endorsing them here, simply showing the wide range of options available for zero-calorie drinks.

Drinks containing calories:
Flavoured green tea (1)
Fruit infusions (fruit teas) (2-4)
Coffee, black (3)
Low calorie fruit squashes (below 10)

Tea with skimmed milk (10)
Beef extract (e.g. Bovril), 1 teaspoon (10)
Yeast extract (e.g. Marmite), 1 tsp (10)
Tea with semi-skimmed milk (15)

And, if your day's calories allow, there are instant 40-calorie hot chocolate drinks available. You just add hot water.

Although this list looks quite short, a few minutes spent at the tea section of your local supermarket will reveal a vast range of flavoured infusions which should satisfy almost all tastes – strawberry, camomile, fennel, peppermint, peach, ginger... the list goes on and on. None of them contains more than 4 calories and placing a mint leaf or two on top will enhance the flavour as well as the appearance and give it that "special" feel. And don't forget stevia if you prefer your drinks sweet!

What of the extra hundred a man is allowed each calorie-restricted day? Well, when I tell you that one glass of fresh orange juice or one banana can account for the whole hundred it doesn't seem that much, does it? He can, of course, opt instead for a couple of squares of chocolate, a chicken drumstick, a small piece of cheese or maybe an apple and tangerine. And since vegetables are generally pretty low in the calorie stakes, a large extra portion of mixed veg may well help to keep his tummy satisfied.

Many of the recipes list salt and pepper as ingredients. This should not be taken as meaning that I think salt is so great that I want you to take in lots of the stuff. Doctors are regularly warning us of the danger to our blood pressure (and therefore our continued wellbeing) of over-consumption of salt and generally I use it very sparingly, if at all. However, it's listed, along with its sidekick pepper, as a seasoning agent to enhance the flavour of food and not to swamp it. In other words, please use salt with due caution.

It is also worth mentioning here that some of the recipes use vegetable or chicken stock. If you are one of those cooks who make their own stock, that's great. However, many of us will reach for the ready-made commercial varieties that come in the form of cubes or gel. If that is so in your case, please take a moment to read on the packaging the recommended dilution with water, since the first ingredient listed in these products is salt –

which means that salt is the most plentiful ingredient. Surprisingly, even the low salt variety still lists salt as the main ingredient! So please don't be tempted to use less water simply because the recipe doesn't use that much.

I haven't included in any of the instructions the need to wash fruit and vegetables because I'm assuming I'm writing for people who are intelligent enough to understand when washing ingredients is necessary. To remind you to do so could be seen as patronising.

To make your restricted calorie day easier to manage, be sure to look at its menu for a day or two ahead so that if a meal involves any shopping or preparation the day before (for instance, if you are wanting a lunch to take to work) you are well prepared.

Where microwave cookers are mentioned, the timings are based on a 750 watt device and if yours differs from this, cooking times will need to be adjusted accordingly. All timings for any cooking, whether frying, baking, grilling, boiling or microwaving, are of course approximate. There's no purpose to be served watching a meal turn black under the grill just to observe the stated times! Appliances vary as does almost everything else in life!

I'm assuming that the reader will already have all the usual cooking utensils. But there are some recipes that require other devices such as a blender. And to make juicing fruit and the occasional vegetable easier I'm also going to suggest a juice extractor, even though it's possible to pulp most things in a blender and sieve them to get the juice you want (which is a messy way of doing it!). A ridged griddle pan, a wok and mortar and pestle are also useful additions to your collection. And don't forget an accurate set of scales: electronic ones can be bought quite cheaply and are indispensible for weighing small quantities.

It will make your program easier if you have a basic collection of ingredients in stock that you can call on as needed in addition to the fresh fruit, vegetables, meat and fish that you have to buy as you need them. The following will be found in the recipes:

mixed spice
nutmeg, grated
nutmeg, ground
ginger, ground

vanilla essence
cinnamon, ground
chilli powder, hot
chilli powder, mild
cumin, ground
garam masala
paprika
coriander, ground
mustard, wholegrain
mustard, strong
soy sauce
vinegar, balsamic
vinegar, cider
stevia extract
salt
lentils, red
lentils, split
olive oil, extra virgin
Tabasco Sauce
sunflower seeds
1 cal olive oil spray
garlic cloves
pepper, black ground
porridge oats
raisins
honey
breadcrumbs
chipotle chilli paste
tamarind paste
vegetable stock cubes
sesame oil
kidney beans, canned
tomatoes, canned chopped
mayonnaise, light
sugar, soft brown
grapefruit segments, canned
mandarin segments, canned
pineapple rings, canned
curry paste

tuna, canned
olives, jar
parmesan cheese, tub

...and a ready supply of ice cubes in the freezer.

Many of these items will no doubt already be on your shelves. Others may be a new taste to you, which will make the diet more of an adventure. It will also help to have some potted herbs on the kitchen windowsill, including mint, coriander, parsley and basil, from which you can freely pick the leaves.

Choosing your favourite crockery and glassware, as well as your finest cutlery, and taking care with presentation, will enhance the experience of your reduced-calorie days.

So that's it – now it's over to you to enjoy the recipes that follow and to lose weight and gain in health as you do.

Bon Appetit!

Daily Menus

A note about presentation

On the following pages the menus displayed cover three meals a day. In order to ensure that each recipe is visible in its entirety I have sometimes found it necessary to start a new page after a recipe that occupies only half a page or so. I thought you'd prefer this rather than having to turn a page with greasy hands midway through a recipe. It may not be an elegant solution but at least it's a practical one!

Menu 1

Breakfast

Grapefruit and Pistachio Delight

1 medium grapefruit
10g (about ½ teaspoon) chopped pistachio nuts
Stevia to taste

- Peel the grapefruit and divide into segments
- Sprinkle with pistachios
- Add Stevia to taste

Reminder: Stevia is very sweet – a third of a teaspoon is as sweet as a whole teaspoon of sugar!

100 calories

Lunch

Cucumber, Orange and Mint Smoothie

1 small apple
½ cucumber
2 small oranges
Mint leaves to taste
Ice cubes (optional)

- Slice the apple and cucumber into thick chunks
- Extract the juice using a juicer
- Squeeze the oranges
- Put all the juice in a blender together with the mint leaves and whisk at high speed for a few seconds
- Add ice cubes to chill

120 calories

Dinner

Tangy Tomato and Mozzarella Salad

5 cherry tomatoes, halved
2 spring onions, trimmed and chopped
½ tablespoon vinegar (preferably balsamic)
15 ml (3 teaspoons) extra virgin olive oil
56g (2oz) mozzarella cheese, cubed
5 sprigs parsley, curly or flat
Several leaves fresh basil
Salt
Ground black pepper

- Put the tomato halves and the spring onions into a large bowl
- Sprinkle the vinegar and oil over the contents of the bowl and toss thoroughly
- Add the cubes of mozzarella and salt and pepper as desired, then toss again
- Cover and leave in the fridge to chill (approx 2 hours)
- Remove 10 minutes before serving
- Finely chop the parsley, shred the basil leaves and sprinkle them over the salad
- Give the salad a final toss

279 calories

Day's total: calories 499

Menu 2

Breakfast

Poached eggs with Crispbread

1 cal cooking spray
2 medium eggs
Salt
Ground black pepper
2 crispbreads

- Coat a microwavable bowl with cooking spray
- Break eggs into bowl, prick yolks
- Spray eggs with cooking spray
- Add salt and pepper to taste
- Cover bowl loosely
- Microwave on high setting for 2 minutes or 1½ minutes if you prefer your yolks softer (based on 750 watt)
- Serve with crispbread slices (e.g. Ryvita)

170 calories

Lunch

Spicy Tomato soup

½ garlic clove, chopped
2 slices root ginger, chopped
½ green chilli, chopped
Pinch ground cumin
½ tsp ground coriander
13g red split lentils
½ tin chopped tomatoes
300ml vegetable stock
½ tbsp tamarind paste
A few coriander leaves
1 tbsp natural yogurt
1 cal cooking oil spray

- Cook the garlic, ginger and chilli in oil spray (about 6 sprays) for 3 minutes to blend flavours
- Add the spices and cook for a further two minutes
- Add the coriander, lentils, tomatoes and stock
- Bring to boil and stir in the tamarind paste
- Simmer for 20 minutes until the lentils are tender
- Transfer to a blender and blend until smooth
- Chop the coriander leaves and fold into the yoghurt
- Stir into the soup and serve

110 calories

Note: please read the information regarding commercial **stock** products if you haven't already done so. You'll find it in the last paragraph on page 19.

Dinner

Ham & Roasted Vegetables

2 slices cooked ham
½ tbsp olive oil
¼ cup beets, cubed
¼ cup onion, cubed
¼ cup parsnip, cubed
¼ cup turnip, cubed
¼ cup courgette, cubed
¼ cup red pepper, cubed
Pinch salt & black pepper

- Preheat oven to 200°C / 390°F / Gas mark 6
- Place cubed vegetables into a bowl
- Sprinkle with olive oil and mix well
- Season with the salt and pepper
- Spread the vegetables out evenly on a baking tray lined with greased foil
- Roast in the hot oven for about 45 minutes, turning halfway through cooking
- Remove from oven when tender and beginning to turn golden
- Serve immediately with the ham slices

210 calories

Day's total: 490 calories

Menu 3

Breakfast

Hot, Cold & Spicy Smoothie

1 tsp honey
½ tsp ground cinnamon
Very tiny sprinkle of hot chilli pepper
Pinch ground nutmeg
1 small banana (6 inches or less) peeled and sliced
1/3 cup kale, chopped
¼ cup spinach
¼ cup water
Ice cubes

- Mix all the above in a blender on high speed until completely smooth
- Add the ice cubes and blend thoroughly
- Pour into a glass and it's ready to drink and savour each mouthful.

108 Calories

Lunch

Tomato and Cabbage Salad with Edamame

Note: Edamame beans are a young soya bean, very popular in Japan. They are becoming increasingly available in the west.

1 teaspoon extra virgin olive oil
1 fl. oz lemon juice
8 cherry tomatoes, halved
½ cup cabbage, chopped
56g (2 oz) Waitrose ready shelled edamame beans
4 olives, halved or sliced

- Cook the edamame beans, as per packet instructions
- Put the cooked beans into a small salad bowl and allow them to cool
- Add the cabbage, cherry tomatoes and olives to the beans
- Drizzle the olive oil and lemon juice over the salad
- Toss the salad to coat evenly

142 Calories

Dinner

Fluffy Ham, Cheese & Tomato Omelette

2 medium eggs
1 teaspoon wholegrain mustard
1 cal olive oil spray
1 slice cooked ham
3 cherry tomatoes
15g (½ oz) grated cheddar cheese
Salt
Ground black pepper
Sprigs of parsley

- Cut the ham into small pieces
- Slice the cherry tomatoes in half
- Separate the egg yolks from the whites
- Beat the yolks with mustard, salt and pepper
- Whisk the egg whites until they stand in soft peaks
- Stir the whites gently into the yolks
- Heat the grill to a high temperature
- Spray an omelette pan with 6 sprays of olive oil spray
- Pour the egg mixture into the pan
- Cook over a medium heat until the underside is golden (about 2 minutes)
- Put the pan under the grill and cook until the top is golden (1 to 2 minutes)
- Sprinkle the ham, cheese and tomatoes over the omelette
- Fold the omelette in half
- Serve, garnished with the parsley

250 calories

Day's total: 500 calories

Menu 4

Breakfast

Banana and Strawberry Smoothie

1 pot (125g) low fat natural yogurt
1/2 small banana
1/2 cup strawberries
1/2 cup water
Ice cubes
Stevia if desired
Mint leaf to decorate

- Blend together banana, strawberries, yoghurt and water on high speed setting until smooth
- If extra sweetness is required, stir in a little Stevia to taste and blend again for a few seconds
- Serve with ice cubes and top with the mint leaf

154 calories

Lunch

Fig and Feta Omelette

¼ cup kale, chopped
½ cup spinach
½ small fig
½ tablespoon spring onions, chopped
5g aubergine, sliced
15g (½ oz) reduced fat feta cheese
1 cal olive oil spray
1 small egg
Pinch ground or grated nutmeg
3 large leaves from a round lettuce
Pinch salt
Ground black pepper

- Place spinach and kale in pan of boiling water and simmer for 4 minutes
- Drain thoroughly and place on kitchen towelling to absorb excess water
- Gently fry spring onion and aubergine in an omelette pan in a few sprays of oil for 3 minutes
- Remove from heat, sprinkle with nutmeg, salt and pepper
- Stir in the spinach and kale
- Pre-heat grill to medium high heat
- Whisk the egg
- Pour the egg over the mixture
- Top with feta cheese and figs. Grill until golden brown.
- Serve on a bed of lettuce

118 calories

Dinner

Spicy Chicken with Tomato, Pepper & Mint Salad

1 small chicken breast (84g/3oz), skinless
¾ tablespoons tamarind purée
1 teaspoon root ginger, grated
¾ teaspoon chilli powder (mild)
Pinch of Stevia
8 cherry tomatoes
Couple of mint leaves, chopped
¼ green chilli, seeded and sliced
1 small sweet yellow pepper
1 small onion
1 large wedge of lemon
Salt
Pepper

- Chop the chicken into chunky pieces
- Place in a bowl and add the tamarind purée, grated ginger, half the chilli powder, pinch of Stevia and salt and pepper
- Mix well and leave to infuse for approximately ten minutes
- Preheat the grill to a high temperature
- Cut the tomatoes in half
- Finely slice the onion and yellow pepper
- Place the tomatoes, pepper and onion in a bowl and add the chilli, mint, the juice of the lemon wedge and the rest of the chilli powder
- Season with salt and pepper to taste
- Push the chicken pieces onto a metal skewer
- Grill the skewered chicken, turning frequently until cooked thoroughly (about ten minutes)
- Place the chicken on a plate and arrange the salad around it admiringly

220 calories

Day's total: 492 calories

Menu 5

Breakfast

Egg & Vegetable Bake

2 large vine tomatoes, halved
1 large mushroom
¼ garlic clove, chopped finely
½ teaspoon olive oil
50g spinach
1 small egg
Salt
Black Pepper

- Heat the oven to 200°C / 390°F / Gas mark 6
- Put tomatoes with mushroom & garlic into an ovenproof dish
- Season with salt and pepper and pour over the oil
- Cook in the oven for 8 minutes
- While it is cooking, pour boiling water over the spinach in a colander to make it wilt
- Tip the spinach onto a piece of kitchen towel. Cover with another piece of kitchen towel and press evenly to remove any water
- After the 10 minutes of baking, remove the dish from the oven and put the spinach in with the other vegetables
- Make a small space in the middle of the vegetables and break the egg into it
- Bake for approximately 8 minutes until the egg is cooked

127 calories

Lunch

Carrot & Coriander Soup

½ onion, chopped
¼ teaspoon ground coriander
2 new potatoes, finely diced
110g carrots, grated
300ml vegetable stock
1 teaspoon coriander leaves, chopped
1 cal olive oil

- Spray a saucepan with 4 sprays 1 cal oil and heat
- Fry the onion for a few minutes until soft
- Mix in the potato and coriander and cook for a further minute
- Add in the carrots and vegetable stock, boil up then reduce heat and cover the pan
- Simmer for about 15 minutes
- Pour the mixture into a blender and add the coriander leaves
- Blend thoroughly until completely smooth
- Reheat if necessary
- Pour into a serving bowl

115 calories

Dinner

Halibut with Barbecue Sauce

½ fillet halibut
1 tablespoon sugar-free apricot jams
½ teaspoon fresh root ginger, finely chopped
2 tablespoons orange juice
2 tablespoons lime juice
½ teaspoon strong mustard
¼ teaspoon cinnamon
¼ teaspoon nutmeg
1 cal olive oil spray
Salt
Ground black pepper

- Put all the ingredients except the fish into a saucepan and boil up
- Reduce the heat and simmer for 5 minutes
- Remove from heat
- Heat the grill to a high setting
- Place the fish on a non-stick grill pan and season with salt and pepper
- Spray fish with olive oil spray (2 sprays)
- Grill for 4 minutes, turn over and brush with the sauce
- Cook for a further 3 minutes
- Brush again with the sauce before serving

239 calories

The remaining sauce can be stored in the fridge for up to a week and used again with other meats or fish

Day's total: 481 calories

Menu 6

Breakfast

Cheese & Tomato Omelette

1 cal olive oil
6 cherry tomatoes
½ small onion, diced
6 fresh basil leaves, chopped
2 small eggs
1 tablespoon grated Parmesan cheese
Salt
Pepper

- Coat a small pan with 5 sprays of 1 cal olive oil and heat gently
- Fry the onion until soft (approximately 4 minutes)
- At the halved tomatoes to the onion and cook for a further 2 – 3 minutes
- Remove from the heat and mix in the basil
- Whisk the eggs with a tablespoon of water and season with salt and pepper
- Heat 4 sprays of 1 cal olive oil in an omelette pan
- Pour in the egg and cook until set
- Sprinkle Parmesan cheese onto one half of the omelette and spread the tomato mixture over the cheese
- Fold the plain half of the omelette over the filled half and cook for a further two minutes until the base is golden brown
- Serve immediately and savour

170 calories

Lunch

Zesty Prawn and Grapefruit Salad

45g fresh prawns, cooked and ready to use
1 small grapefruit, segmented
2 large leaves from a round lettuce
1 tablespoon low fat mayonnaise
A few drops of Tabasco sauce
6 fresh mint leaves, chopped
Salt
Pepper

- Spoon the mayonnaise into a cup and season with Tabasco sauce, salt and pepper to taste
- Place the salad leaves overlapping in the middle of a plate
- Arrange the prawns and grapefruit segments on centre of the lettuce
- Sprinkle the mint leaves on top
- Spoon the spicy mayonnaise onto the side of the plate to use as a dip

87 calories

Dinner

Spicy Chicken Breast

1 skinless chicken breast fillet
2 sprigs of parsley, finely chopped
Pinch of cumin
Pinch of coriander
1 cal olive oil spray
125ml vegetable stock
Pepper
Pinch of chilli powder (optional)

Side salad:

1 cup lettuce
6 radishes
1 tomato quartered
6 slices cucumber

- Pre-heat oven to 200^0C / 390^0F / Gas mark 6
- Use a sharp knife to make 3 small cuts in the chicken
- In a bowl, mix the herbs and spices well
- Cover the chicken breast with the mixture, pushing some of it into the cuts
- Spray twice with the olive oil
- Pour the stock into a small, shallow oven dish
- Carefully transfer the chicken fillet onto the dish
- Cook for 20 minutes. Make sure the chicken is cooked thoroughly and that the coating is golden brown before removing
- Slice the chicken and serve with the side salad

240 calories

Day's total: 497 calories

Menu 7

Breakfast

Grape Booster

1 cup seedless grapes, red
½ cup seedless grapes, green
¼ cup purple grape juice
1 teaspoon lime juice
½ teaspoon root ginger, chopped
Ice cubes

- Put the grapes, juices, ginger and ice cubes into a blender and mix thoroughly
- Serve in a tall glass

123 Calories

Lunch

Filled Mushrooms

3 large mushrooms, cleaned and hollowed out
½ tablespoon tomatoes, chopped
½ tablespoon red peppers, chopped
½ tablespoon olives, chopped
½ fresh garlic clove
¼ tablespoon fresh parsley, finely chopped
¼ teaspoon fresh oregano leaves, chopped
Fresh ground black pepper, to taste
¼ teaspoon fresh lemon juice
½ teaspoon olive oil
30g feta cheese, crumbled
3 sprigs parsley to garnish

- Lightly grease a baking tray or line with foil
- Clean the mushrooms with a damp piece of kitchen towel
- Remove the stalks and hollow out the heads
- Mix the tomatoes, peppers, olives, parsley, oregano, lemon and olive oil in a bowl
- Crush the garlic into the mix and stir well
- Fill the mushroom heads equally and put them on the baking tray
- Cook for approximately 20 minutes or until the smell drives you mad with anticipation
- Serve on a plate with a sprig of parsley to garnish each one

94 Calories

Dinner

Spicy Fish Dish

125g fillet white fish
1 tablespoon chilli pesto
½ tablespoon breadcrumbs

½ tablespoon Parmesan cheese, grated
125g green beans, trimmed
½ teaspoon of butter
½ lemon, sliced in wedges
Salt
Pepper

- Heat the oven to 200⁰C / 390⁰F Gas mark 6
- Put the fillet on a greased baking tray
- Season with salt and pepper and coat with chilli pesto
- Mix the breadcrumbs with the Parmesan cheese and sprinkle on the fish
- Bake for about 10 minutes until the fish is cooked and the topping bubbles
- Meanwhile, boil or steam the beans until tender then stir in the butter and the juice of one lemon wedge
- Arrange the fish on a plate with the beans and decorate with the remainder of the lemon wedges

Note: adjust the amount of chilli pesto to suit your own taste. It can be quite fiery!

258 calories

Day's calorie total: 475

Menu 8

Breakfast

Fruity Delight

1 small pot fat-free peach yogurt
90g pineapple chunks, canned or fresh
75g raspberries, fresh or frozen

- Layer a sundae glass with yoghurt, pineapple and raspberries, with a raspberry on top of the yoghurt
- And that's it! Easy peasy!

109 calories

Lunch

Tasty Green Veggie Soup

3 sticks celery, chopped
¼ leek, sliced
50g spinach
300ml vegetable stock
1 cal olive oil spray
½ tablespoon fat-free yoghurt

- Use 5 sprays of olive oil to coat a frying pan
- Fry the leek and celery on a gentle heat for approximately 5 minutes, until the leeks are soft
- Add the stock and cook for 25 minutes on a low heat
- Mix in the spinach and continue to cook for 5 minutes
- Pour the mixture into a blender and liquidize
- Swirl in the yoghurt and serve

80 calories

Dinner

Beefy Chilli Stir Fry

50g fillet steak, thinly sliced
½ red chilli, deseeded and chopped
2 teaspoons rice wine vinegar
1 piece root ginger, finely chopped
1 clove garlic, crushed
2 teaspoons light soy sauce
2 spring onions, trimmed and sliced
100g broccoli, chopped into small pieces
100g courgettes, diced
100g pak choi (Chinese cabbage), chopped
1 teaspoon sesame oil

- Stir the chilli, ginger and garlic into the soy sauce and rice wine vinegar
- Put the beef slices into the sauce mix
- Heat the sesame oil in a wok until it smokes
- Lift the beef from the sauce and cook with the courgettes and spring onion for 1 minute
- Add the broccoli and pak choi to the wok and cook for another 2 minutes, stirring continuously until cooked
- Pour in the sauce and stir well
- Serve immediately

227 calories

Day's total 416 calories

Menu 9

Breakfast

Pear Peach & Strawberry Cocktail

½ pear, peeled and chopped
½ peach, stoned and chopped
100g strawberries, halved
Large wedge of lime
Ice cube

- Put the pear. Peach and strawberries into a blender
- Squeeze the juice of the lime on top
- Add the ice cube
- Blend until smooth
- Pour into a glass and drink

98 Calories

Lunch

Honeyed Chicken Stir-Fry with Noodles

1 small skinless chicken breast
4 teaspoons sweet chilli stir fry sauce
1½ teaspoons clear honey
1" cube fresh root ginger, grated
1 clove garlic, finely chopped
1 tablespoon water
2 spring onions, trimmed and thinly sliced
30g precooked rice noodles
Salt
Pepper

- In a cup, mix the sweet chilli stir-fry sauce, honey, ginger, garlic and water
- Dice the chicken

- Heat a wok and dry-fry the chicken pieces for a few seconds to colour them
- Pour the honey mixture over the chicken and stir
- Season with salt and pepper
- Stir-fry over a medium heat for about 10 minutes
- Add the precooked noodles for the last 3 minutes
- Serve with the sliced spring onion scattered over the top

200 calories

Dinner

Lemon and Parsley Haddock with Green Beans

1 fresh haddock fillet
Juice and grated zest of ½ lemon
56g (2 oz) breadcrumbs
6 sprigs parsley, finely chopped
1 tomato, halved
1 cal olive oil spray
1 cup trimmed green beans
Salt
Pepper

- Preheat the oven to 170⁰C / 340⁰F / Gas mark 3- 4
- Mix the breadcrumbs, lemon zest, parsley and lemon juice
- Add salt and pepper to taste
- Use the breadcrumb mix to coat the fish
- Spray a baking tray with 2 sprays 1 cal olive oil
- Put the coated fish and tomato halves on the baking tray
- Spray twice with 1 cal olive oil
- Cook in the oven for 20 minutes
- While it is cooking, steam or boil the beans
- Serve the fish with the cooked green beans
- Bon appétit!

200 Calories

Day's total: 498 calories

Menu 10

Breakfast

Banana and Ginger Smoothie

1 extra small banana (below 6 inches)
¼ teaspoon ginger root, grated
1 tablespoon coconut milk
¼ cup apple juice
Ice cubes

- Put all the ingredients in a blender
- Blend thoroughly
- Serve in a glass
- Simples!

150 Calories

Lunch

Courgette and Chive Omelette

2 small eggs
1 courgette, finely diced
1 teaspoon chives, chopped
1 cal olive oil
Salt
Pepper
- Whisk the eggs thoroughly
- Add the courgette and chives
- Season with salt and pepper
- Spray a frying pan with 3 sprays olive oil and heat on a medium setting
- Pour in the egg mixture
- Cook until firm on one side then flip over and cook until the base is golden brown
- Serve immediately

127 calories

Dinner

Chilli Chicken Stir Fry

75g chicken breast strips, skinless
1 tablespoon spicy chipotle chilli paste
150g vegetable stir fry mix
1 cal olive oil spray

- Mix the chipotle chilli paste thoroughly with the chicken strips
- Leave to marinate for 1 hour
- Spray a wok with 2 sprays of olive oil and fry the chicken, stirring continuously for 3 to 5 minutes until completely cooked
- Remove the chicken and place on one side
- Spray the wok with 2 more sprays of oil
- Stir fry the vegetable mix for about 2 minutes on a medium heat
- Stir in the chicken whilst heating for a further 3 minutes
- Serve up!

Note: as with any chilli product, the chilli paste should be adjusted to your own taste. It can be quite fiery!

180 Calories

Days total: 457 calories

Menu 11

Breakfast

Spicy Apple Porridge

1 small apple, cubed
1 teaspoon vanilla essence
1 teaspoon cinnamon
A pinch of mixed spice
1 teaspoon raisins
¼ cup water
10g porridge oats
60ml semi-skimmed milk
Stevia to taste (optional)

- Place the cubed apples in a pan with the vanilla essence, cinnamon, mixed spice, raisins and ¼ cup of water
- Put the lid on the pan and simmer, stirring occasionally for about 10 minutes
- Remove from heat and leave covered
- Mix the oats with the semi-skimmed milk and salt in a large, microwavable bowl
- Cook on full power for 2 minutes
- Pour the porridge into a serving bowl and add the stewed, spicy apple. Leave in the centre or swirl in gently
- Sweeten with Stevia to taste

130 calories

Lunch

Salmon and Cream Cheese Toasty Munch

1 slice wholemeal bread
1 tablespoon low-fat cream cheese
28g (1 oz) sliced smoked salmon
1 small red onion, sliced

56g (2 oz) alfalfa and radish shoots

- Toast the bread on both sides
- Spread the cream cheese on top of the toast
- Arrange the salmon, onions slices and alfalfa & radish shoots over the top
- Eat and enjoy!

Calories: 179

Dinner

Vegetable Stir Fry

1 cal olive oil spray
4 spring onions, thinly sliced
1 tablespoon root ginger, chopped finely
½ small yellow pepper, sliced thinly
½ small red pepper, sliced thinly
1 leaf choi sum., shredded
56g (2 oz) bean sprouts
1 clove garlic, chopped
56g (2 oz) sugar snaps peas
1 tablespoon sesame oil
2 tablespoons soy sauce

- Coat a wok well with olive oil spray 6 sprays
- Fry the onions, ginger and garlic gently until soft (about 3 minutes)
- Add the peppers and sugar snap peas and continue cooking for 3 more minutes
- Add the choi sum and bean sprouts, together with the soy sauce and sesame oil
- Stir fry for a further 2 minutes
- Serve straight away

Calories 191

Day's total: 500 calories

Menu 12

Breakfast

Poached Egg with Watercress and Tomatoes

1 large egg
6 cherry tomatoes, diced
30g (1oz) watercress, chopped
1 tsp sunflower seeds
1 teaspoon coriander, chopped

- Boil a small pan of water
- Remove from heat and swirl the water rapidly with a wooden spoon
- Break the egg into the centre of the swirling water
- Cook for about two minutes or until the egg is firm
- Remove egg with a slotted spoon and allow the water to drain away
- Place the sunflower seeds dry into a heavy-bottomed pan or skillet
- Heat over a medium heat for about 2 minutes or until golden brown, keeping the pan moving to avoid burning the seeds
- Mix the seeds with the watercress and tomatoes and arrange on a plate
- Place the egg on the salad and top with coriander

108 calories

Lunch

Potato, Onion & Greens Soup

¼ bunch spring onions, chopped
1 cal olive oil spray
1 small potato, peeled and diced
300ml vegetable stock
70g watercress, spinach and rocket salad
Pepper
Sprig of parsley
Slice of crispbread

- Coat the bottom of a small saucepan with 5 sprays of 1 cal olive oil spray and heat
- Fry the chopped spring onions gently until tender
- Put in the potato and cook with the onions for 2 minutes
- Pour in the stock, add a little black pepper and cook until the potato is soft and beginning to crumble
- Stir in the salad leaves and continue to cook gently for a further minute
- Pour into a blender and liquidize thoroughly
- Serve, topped with a sprig of parsley
- Enjoy with a crispbread slice

112 calories

Dinner

Grilled Lamb Chop Special

2 lamb loin chops (about 190g total)
¼ of small orange pepper, diced
1 teaspoon chopped red onion
1 cup baby spinach leaves
Wedge of lemon
1 cal olive oil spray

Dressing:
    ¼ teaspoon grated lemon rind
    1 tablespoon clear honey
    ¼ tablespoon fresh thyme, chopped
    ¼ clove garlic, finely chopped
    ½ teaspoon grain mustard
    Salt & Ground pepper

- Preheat the grill to a medium level
- Put the dressing ingredients into a medium sized bowl and mix well
- Remove 1 teaspoon of the dressing and put in a salad bowl for later
- Coat the chops thoroughly in the bowl with the remainder of the dressing and leave to marinate for about 10 minutes
- Spray the grill pan with 3 sprays of olive oil
- Place the chops on the grill pan
- Grill gently, turning occasionally until cooked to your taste (about 10 minutes for medium rare)
- In the bowl with the teaspoon of dressing put the orange pepper, onion and spinach leaves and mix well
- Put the dressed salad on a plate and place the chops on top
- Put the lemon wedge on the side of the plate and your delicious meal is ready!

270 calories

Day's total: 490 calories

Menu 13

Breakfast

Fruit & Vegetable Juice

½ medium carrot
2 sticks celery
1 apple
1 tomato
1 thin slice root ginger
Sprig of mint

- Cut all ingredients except mint into small pieces
- Put pieces into juicer and switch on
- Collect the juice in a glass
- Pop in the sprig of mint
- Done!

75 calories

Lunch

Chicken Liver Lunch

50g chicken liver
150g green beans
¼ teaspoon olive oil
4 thin spring onions, sliced

For the Dressing:
    1 tsp olive oil
    1 tbsp soy sauce
    ½ teaspoon cider vinegar

- Steam the green beans until tender.
- Meanwhile, preheat the grill on a medium setting
- Press the liver flat and place on a grill tray
- Drizzle ¼ tsp olive oil over the liver
- Grill the liver for 2 minutes on each side
- Mix the ingredients for the dressing in a small bowl
- Stir in the spring onion and beans
- Slice the liver finely and stir into the salad
- Spoon onto a plate and eat

Total: 183 calories

Dinner

Mediterranean Beef

75g lean beef steak, thinly sliced
¼ garlic clove, sliced
¼ onion, sliced
1 cal olive oil spray
100g (3½ oz) canned chopped tomatoes
¼ yellow pepper, thinly sliced
Pinch chopped rosemary
2 olives, chopped
84g (3 oz) slice of precooked polenta

- Spray a saucepan with 4 sprays olive oil
- Fry the onion and garlic for about 5 minutes until the onion is starting to brown
- Add the beef, tomatoes, pepper and rosemary and stir well
- Simmer gently in the covered pan, stirring occasionally, until the beef is cooked (about 15 minutes)
- Preheat the grill to medium
- If the mixture becomes too dry, add a little boiling water
- Add the olives and stir again
- Grill the polenta for about 3 minutes each side during the last six minutes of the beef cooking
- Place the polenta beside the beef mix on a plate and serve hot. Buona appetita!

225 calories

Day's total: 483 calories

Menu 14

Breakfast

Pineapple and Cottage Cheese Toasty

1 slice wholemeal bread
1 oz cottage cheese
1 teaspoon cinnamon
1 slice pineapple

- Preheat the grill to a medium heat
- Toast the bread lightly on both sides
- Spread the cottage cheese evenly over the toast
- Sprinkle with the cinnamon
- Place the pineapple on top
- Put the toasty under the grill
- Grill until the cheese begins to brown

128 Calories

Lunch

Greek Salad

1 plum tomato, chopped
1 oz low fat feta cheese
½ small yellow pepper, chopped
½ red onion, chopped
¼ cucumber, diced
3 large pitted olives, halved

Dressing:
    ½ tablespoon balsamic vinegar
    ¼ tablespoon olive oil
    Salt
    Ground pepper

- Place all the prepared salad vegetables in a bowl
- Crumble the feta cheese into the salad
- Pour the vinegar and olive oil into a small lidded container, add a small amount of salt and pepper and shake vigorously
- Pour the dressing onto the salad and mix well before serving

Note: if you increase the quantities of the dressing you can store the remainder in the fridge for another salad on another day.

159 calories

Dinner

Baked Vegetables with Salmon

1 salmon fillet
1 very small garlic clove, crushed
1 tablespoon extra virgin olive oil
½ small tomato, chopped
1 cup spinach
¼ cup mushrooms, chopped
3 large leaves from a round lettuce

- Preheat the oven to 190° C / 375° F / Gas mark 5
- Use a little of the olive oil to grease a small baking dish
- Place the salmon on the baking dish, skin underneath
- Put the rest of the olive oil into a small bowl, add the garlic, tomato, spinach and mushrooms, and mix thoroughly
- Cover the salmon with the mixture
- Cook for about 20 minutes
- Serve on a bed of lettuce

188 calories

Day's total: 475 calories

Menu 15

Breakfast

Scrummy Scrambled Egg

1 large egg
1 tablespoon water
¼ cup onion, chopped
¼ cup firm tomato, diced
4 good sized basil leaves, chopped finely
2 tablespoons grated low fat cheddar cheese
Salt to taste
Ground pepper to taste
1 cal olive oil spray
2 sprigs fresh parsley

- Beat egg and water in a bowl
- Coat a small frying pan with 4 sprays of 1 cal spray and heat
- Add onion and cook gently whilst stirring until soft and translucent
- Mix in the diced tomato, chopped basil leaves, salt and pepper
- Cook for a further minute
- Pour the beaten egg into the pan and stir continuously until the egg is cooked
- Transfer to a plate scatter with the grated cheese
- Decorate with the parsley and savour slowly!

136 calories

Lunch

Tuna Salad

½ small can tuna chunks in brine
1 large egg
4 cherry tomatoes, halved
3 large lettuce leaves, shredded
Salt
Pepper

- Hard-boil the egg in boiling water (about 10 minutes). Drain and leave to cool
- Put the shredded lettuce and the tomatoes in a bowl with the tuna and mix together
- When the egg has cooled down, shell and chop it
- Stir the egg pieces into the rest of the salad
- Season and serve

185 calories

Dinner

Chicken & Mushroom Broth, Thai Style

50g ready cooked chicken, shredded
250ml chicken stock
¼ tablespoon Thai red curry paste
¼ tablespoon Thai fish sauce
½ lime, zest and juice
½ teaspoon sugar
25g mushrooms, sliced
2 spring onions, chopped

- Heat the stock in a medium sized saucepan
- Add the curry paste, sugar, fish sauce, lime juice and zest
- When boiling, add in the mushrooms and spring onion pieces
- Cover the pan and simmer the mixture for 2 minutes
- Add the chicken and stir well
- Serve in your favourite bowl

179 calories

Day's total: 500 calories

Menu 16

Breakfast

Tropical Shake

125g tropical fruit, frozen
1 tablespoon oats
100ml orange juice
100ml soya milk

- Put all the ingredients into a blender
- Blend thoroughly until completely smooth
- Serve in a tall glass

209 calories

Lunch

Hot Toddy

½ lemon
Small piece fresh root ginger, finely sliced
3 teaspoons honey
300 ml boiling water

- Cut the lemon into two pieces and squeeze the juice of one piece into a mug
- Cut the other piece of lemon into slices
- Put the lemon slices, ginger and honey in the mug
- Add the boiling water
- Allow 5 minutes for infusion
- It's ready to drink. Cheers!

69 calories

Note: If you have a cold, this drink is very soothing. If you don't, it's delicious anyway.

Dinner

Mediterranean Chicken

112g (4oz) diced chicken breast
½ garlic clove, sliced
100g (3½oz) rocket
2 sticks celery, finely chopped
1 teaspoon basil, chopped
½ lemon
¼ onion, chopped
6 cherry tomatoes, halved
1 cal olive oil

- Spray a frying pan with 3 sprays of olive oil
- Fry the chicken gently until cooked (about 10 minutes) and turn off the heat
- Put the garlic, rocket, celery, basil and onion into a blender and squeeze in the lemon juice
- Blend thoroughly
- Pour the mixture over the chicken, add the tomatoes and stir well
- Serve while hot

203 cal

Day's total: 481

Menu 17

Breakfast

Toasty Spicy Slice

1 slice of white bread
1 teaspoon peanut butter
1 tablespoon natural fat-free yoghurt
1 small banana, sliced
Small pinch of cinnamon
Small pinch of ground ginger
Small pinch of mixed spice

- Mix the peanut butter and yoghurt thoroughly in a bowl
- Toast the bread
- Spread the mixture on the toast and arrange the slices of banana on top
- Season with the cinnamon, ginger and mixed spice
- Eat slowly, relishing each mouthful

163 calories

Lunch

Smoked Salmon and Radishes with Poppy Seed Dressing

50g smoked salmon
¼ tablespoon poppy seeds
Juice and zest of ½ orange
½ teaspoon cider vinegar
½ teaspoon olive oil
A couple of drops of sesame oil
8 radishes, finely sliced
1 spring onion, finely sliced
black pepper
1 slice of crispbread

- In a bowl, mix thoroughly the poppy seeds, vinegar, sesame oil, olive oil, orange zest and juice and black pepper
- Place the salmon in another bowl and add the sliced radishes and spring onion
- Pour the dressing over the salmon and mix everything carefully until the salmon is completely coated
- Leave to marinate for 10 minutes
- Place the salmon on a plate and pour over any remaining dressing
- Serve up with two slices of crispbread

120 calories

Dinner

Chicken Tandoori

2 small chicken thighs, skinless
Juice of ¼ lemon
½ tsp paprika
½ red onion, finely chopped
1 cal olive oil
1 garlic & coriander poppadom (accompaniment)

Marinade:
  50ml fat-free Greek yogurt
  Pinch ground cumin
  Small piece of ginger, grated
  Pinch garam masala
  ½ garlic clove, crushed
  Pinch chilli powder
  Pinch turmeric

- In a bowl, mix together the paprika, lemon juice and onion
- With a sharp knife make 2 slits in each chicken thigh
- Coat the thighs well with the juice and leave them in the bowl to steep for 10 minutes
- Take a jug, put all the marinade ingredients into it, and stir thoroughly
- Pour the marinade onto the chicken thighs and coat them well with the mixture
- Cover the bowl and refrigerate for 1 hour
- Heat the grill to medium
- Put the chicken pieces on a lightly oiled baking tray and spray a couple of times with the olive oil
- Grill them for 8 minutes before turning over and grilling the other side for a further 8 minutes
- Check that the chicken is thoroughly cooked before serving
- Serve with the poppadom

206 calories

Day's total: 489 calories

Menu 18

Breakfast

Sharp and Sweet Fruit Salad

½ tablespoon lemon juice
1 small apple, cubed
½ cup strawberries, chopped
75g canned mandarin orange segments in juice
50g canned grapefruit segments in juice
Stevia to taste (optional)

- Put the apple and strawberries into a serving bowl and coat well with the lemon juice
- Stir in the grapefruit and mandarin segments with their juice
- If the flavour is too sharp for your taste, add a little Stevia

Note: Leaving the cans of grapefruit and mandarin in the fridge overnight will chill them nicely for a refreshing summer breakfast.

130 calories

Lunch

Cauliflower and Onion Soup

300ml vegetable stock
1 tablespoon lemon juice
1 small cauliflower, separated into florets
1 cal olive oil
6 spring onions, trimmed & chopped
Small pinch nutmeg
Large pinch black pepper
Sprig of parsley

- Put the stock and lemon juice in a pan and heat until boiling

- Lower the heat to medium and cook the cauliflower in the liquid for 8 to 10 minutes until soft
- Cover and leave
- Heat the oil in a frying pan on a medium heat and fry the chopped onions for 4 – 5 minutes
- Stir the cooked spring onions into the pan with the cauliflower
- Pour the contents of the pan into a blender and blend until smooth
- Add the pepper and nutmeg and stir
- Serve with a garnish of parsley

87 calories

Dinner

Courgette, Lentil and Feta Salad

500g baby courgettes
1 tsp olive oil
2 tablespoons cooked puy lentils (canned)
30g feta cheese, cut into small chunks
¾ teaspoon lemon zest
1 tablespoon mint leaves, shredded
Pinch of salt

- Cut the courgettes lengthwise into long batons
- Put them on a plate, add a pinch of salt and turn well until all the batons are oily
- Place the batons onto a hot, ridged griddle
- Cook until the batons have brown stripes on both sides. Turn while cooking
- Place the courgettes in a bowl and add the lentils, feta cheese and lemon zest
- Mix thoroughly
- Stir in the shredded mint leaves and serve

276 calories

Day's total: 493 calories

Menu 19

Breakfast

Banana Muffins

4 oz self-raising flour
Generous pinch of salt
1 medium banana, mashed
1 oz sugar
1 oz apple sauce
1 small egg
A few drops of vanilla essence

- Preheat oven to 170°C / 350°F / Gas mark 3-4
- Grease muffin tray or muffin cups
- Put flour and salt into a mixing bowl
- Into another bowl, place the mashed banana, sugar, vanilla and egg and beat well, then stir in the apple sauce
- Scoop the banana mixture into the flour and mix well
- Divide the mixture evenly into six muffin cups
- Place in the oven and bake for 20 minutes. If a toothpick pushed into the centre emerges clean, the muffins are cooked
- Allow to cool before eating
- Eat 2 and store the rest

150 calories

This recipe makes 6 muffins. The rest may be stored in an airtight storage box. The flavour improves overnight so making them the night before will mean you have a ready breakfast when you get up.

Lunch

Refreshing Raspberry Fizz

75g raspberries
250 ml sparkling water
Small wedge of lemon
1 teaspoon honey

- Wash raspberries and liquidize them in a blender.
- Pour into a jug and add the sparkling water and squeeze in the lemon juice.
- Stir gently.
- Sieve the mixture to get rid of seeds.
- Stir in the honey.

60 calories

Dinner

Salmon fishcake with Petits Pois
(Makes 4 fishcakes but you can refrigerate the three uneaten ones
to eat on other days.)
120g (4 oz) smoked salmon
500g (18 oz) potatoes (floury, e.g. Maris Piper)
4 spring onions
1 medium egg
1 tablespoon light mayonnaise
2 tablespoons fresh chopped parsley
1 sprig parsley for garnish
Salt to taste
Ground black pepper
5 drops Tabasco sauce (optional)
15g (½ oz) butter
60g breadcrumbs

- Peel and boil the potatoes until soft.
- Finely chop the salmon.
- Trim and chop the spring onions.
- Drain the potatoes and return them to the pan.
- Mash the potatoes thoroughly and mix in the spring onions.
- Put the mixture into a large bowl and spread it so that it cools quickly.
- Separate the egg and beat the yolk and mayonnaise into the mash.
- Fold in the salmon and parsley then add the seasonings.
- Divide the mixture into four equal parts and shape into fishcakes.
- Beat the egg white then brush it over the fishcakes before coating them in breadcrumbs.
- Melt the butter in a small frying pan on a medium heat and cook one fishcake gently until golden and crispy (about 5 minutes each side).
- Serve with ½ cup of cooked frozen petits pois

290 calories

Day's total: 500 calories

Menu 20

Breakfast

Boiled Egg with Asparagus Fingers

1 large egg
1 cal olive oil spray
12g dried breadcrumbs
Pinch of chilli powder
Pinch of paprika
4 asparagus spears
Salt

- Fry the breadcrumbs gently in 4 sprays of hot oil until golden blown
- Mix in the chilli, paprika and salt and place to one side
- Place the asparagus in a saucepan of boiling water, add a little salt and cook until tender (about 5 minutes)
- While the asparagus is cooking, cook the egg in a pan of boiling water for approximately 5 minutes
- Put the egg in an egg cup in the middle of a plate and arrange the drained asparagus around it
- Sprinkle the crumbs over the asparagus and your breakfast is ready

145 calories

Lunch

Minty Pineapple and Grapefruit

½ tin pineapple rings, drained
180g canned red grapefruit, drained
1 tablespoon soft brown sugar
1 tablespoons mint leaves

- Arrange the fruit tastefully in a serving bowl
- Pound the mint and sugar together using a mortar and pestle
- Once they are completely blended, sprinkle the minty sugar over the fruit and enjoy the mingled flavours

168 calories

Dinner

Vegetable Chilli

½ clove garlic, crushed
½ red chilli, chopped
¼ teaspoon ground cumin
65g mushrooms, quartered
100g canned kidney beans
100g canned chopped tomatoes
40g green beans, trimmed and sliced
50ml water
1 teaspoon low-fat crème fraîche
Piece of crusty bread
1 cal olive oil spray

- Spray a frying pan four times with the olive oil and heat
- Put in the garlic and the chilli and fry for 2 minutes
- Add the mushrooms and cumin and cook for a further 3 minutes
- Pour in the tomatoes, kidney beans and water

- Simmer for 10 minutes, stirring occasionally
- Mix in the green beans and cook for five more minutes until the sauce thickens and the beans are soft
- Pour into a serving bowl, top with crème fraîche and enjoy with 2 slices of crispy wheat crispbreads

181 calories

Day's total: 494 calories

Meals Index

From here you can mix and match according to your own tastes. The calorie count for each meal is given in brackets. The meals marked with an asterisk (*) are suitable for vegetarians.

Breakfasts	Menu
Grapefruit and Pistachio Delight (100) *	1
Poached eggs with Crispbread (170) *	2
Hot, Cold & Spicy Smoothie (108) *	3
Banana and Strawberry Smoothie (154) *	4
Egg & Vegetable bake (127) *	5
Cheese & Tomato Omelette (170) *	6
Grape Booster (123) *	7
Fruity Delight (109) *	8
Pear Peach & Strawberry Cocktail (98) *	9
Banana and Ginger Smoothie (150) *	10
Spicy Apple Porridge (130) *	11
Poached Egg with Watercress and Tomatoes (108) *	12
Fruit & Vegetable Juice (75) *	13
Pineapple and Cottage Cheese Toasty (128) *	14
Scrummy Scrambled Egg (136) *	15
Tropical Shake (209) *	16
Toasty Spicy Slice (163) *	17
Sharp and Sweet Fruit Salad (130) *	18
Banana Muffins (150) *	19
Boiled Egg with Asparagus Fingers (145) *	20

Lunches   Menu

Cucumber, Orange and Mint Smoothie (120) *	**1**
Spicy Tomato soup (110) *	**2**
Tomato and Cabbage Salad with Edamame (142) *	**3**
Fig and Feta Omelette (118) *	**4**
Carrot & Coriander Soup (115) *	**5**
Zesty Prawn and Grapefruit Salad (87)	**6**
Filled Mushrooms (94) *	**7**
Tasty Green Veggie Soup (80) *	**8**
Honeyed Chicken Stir-Fry with Noodles (200)	**9**
Courgette and Chive Omelette (127) *	**10**
Salmon and Cream Cheese Toasty Munch (179)	**11**
Potato, Onion & Greens Soup (140) *	**12**
Chicken Liver Lunch (183	**13**
)Greek Salad (159) *	**14**
Tuna Salad (185)	**15**
Hot Toddy (69) *	**16**
Smoked Salmon and Radishes with Poppy Seed Dressing (140)	**17**
Cauliflower and Onion Soup (87) *	**18**
Refreshing Raspberry Fizz (60) *	**19**
Minty Pineapple and Grapefruit (168) *	**20**

Dinners

Menu

Tangy Tomato and Mozzarella Salad (279) *	1
Ham & Roasted Vegetables (210)	2
Fluffy Ham, Cheese & Tomato Omelette (250) *	3
Spicy Chicken with Tomato, Pepper & Mint Salad (215)	4
Halibut with Barbecue Sauce (239)	5
Spicy Chicken Breast (240)	6
Spicy Fish Dish (258)	7
Beefy Chilli Stir Fry (227)	8
Lemon and Parsley Haddock with Green Beans (200)	9
Chilli Chicken Stir Fry (180)	10
Vegetable Stir Fry (191) *	11
Grilled Lamb Chop Special (270)	12
Mediterranean Beef (225)	13
Baked Vegetables with Salmon (188)	14
Chicken & Mushroom Broth, Thai Style (179)	15
Mediterranean Chicken (203)	16
Chicken Tandoori (206)	17
Courgette, Lentil and Feta Salad (276) *	18
Salmon fishcake with Petits Pois (290)	19
Vegetable Chilli (181) *	20

Made in the USA
Lexington, KY
03 April 2013